Distribution, publication, and copying in any form are prohibited and subject to damages.

TEN HYPNOSES

Copying, publishing, and sharing with third parties are only permitted with the written consent of the author. Please observe the notes on copyright and usage.

Distribution, publication, and copying in any form are prohibited and subject to damages.

Copying, publishing, and sharing with third parties are only permitted with the written consent of the author. Please observe the notes on copyright and usage.

Distribution, publication, and copying in any form are prohibited and subject to damages.

Ingo Michael Simon

TEN HYPNOSES

32
OVERCOMING LONELINESS

Copying, publishing, and sharing with third parties are only permitted with the written consent of the author. Please observe the notes on copyright and usage.

Distribution, publication, and copying in any form are prohibited and subject to damages.

© 2024 Ingo Michael Simon
All rights reserved.
Independently published
www.ingosimon.com

Important Notes for Urgent Attention:

The contents of this book are based on the practical experiences of the author with hypnosis applications and psychotherapy in a trance state. Although the author has strived for the utmost care, errors or misunderstandings in the presentation cannot be completely excluded. Therapeutic work with people and the application of hypnosis are solely the responsibility of the hypnotist. It cannot be ruled out that parts of this book may be misunderstood or that the application of a presented procedure may cause an undesirable reaction in the client. The author also assumes no co-responsibility if work with a client is carried out with reference to the statements in this book.

The Author:

Ingo Michael Simon studied psychology and education and is a hypnotherapist with practices in southwestern Germany and Switzerland. With the help of hypnosis-supported psychotherapy, he primarily treats people with persistent psychological conditions. His practice focuses on anxiety disorders, pathological compulsions, and psychosomatic illnesses. His therapeutic offerings mainly include classical and modern hypnosis applications and the dreamland therapy he developed himself.

Copying, publishing, and sharing with third parties are only permitted with the written consent of the author. Please observe the notes on copyright and usage.

Distribution, publication, and copying in any form are prohibited and subject to damages.

INTRODUCTION — 6

COPYRIGHT AND USAGE — 8

HYPNOSIS 1 — 10

HYPNOSIS 2 — 14

HYPNOSIS 3 — 18

HYPNOSIS 4 — 22

HYPNOSIS 5 — 26

HYPNOSIS 6 — 31

HYPNOSIS 7 — 35

HYPNOSIS 8 — 39

HYPNOSIS 9 — 44

HYPNOSIS 0 — 49

ALL TITLES IN THE SERIES — 55

Copying, publishing, and sharing with third parties are only permitted with the written consent of the author. Please observe the notes on copyright and usage.

Introduction

The series "Ten Hypnoses" is very well known in Germany, Austria, and Switzerland as a collection of texts for therapeutic work and is used by numerous psychotherapeutic practices, doctors, therapists, coaches, and other helping professionals. I am pleased to now be able to offer these texts in other countries as well.

Most therapists have their own methods for inducing and deepening trance as well as for exiting trance. Therefore, I have focused on the main part of the hypnosis. The texts in this book can be integrated as the main part into any hypnosis process. The texts in this collection use various hypnosis techniques. I will not explain these in detail, as I assume that users have the appropriate training. It is also not necessary to understand the exact structure or functioning of the different parts. The texts can simply be read aloud, and they will have their effect.

Decide for yourself which text best suits your client or patient at any given time. You can also combine passages from different texts. It is not about using all ten hypnoses in sequence. It is a selection of possibilities.

I want to emphasize that books cannot replace therapy. Psychotherapy or other therapeutic treatments involve much more. A careful diagnosis is the necessary basis for deciding on the use of methods, including whether hypnosis or one of my texts should be used. Even in this case, preparatory discussions, follow-up discussions during the session, and of course, a therapeutic concept for the sequence of sessions and the content approaches are essential parts of therapy. This cannot and should not be achieved with a collection of texts.

In any case, I wish you much success in your work and I am pleased if my text templates can contribute in a small way.

Ingo Michael Simon

Copyright and Usage

Copying, publishing, and sharing with third parties is prohibited and only permitted with the written consent of the author. Please observe the following copyright and usage guidelines.

This work has been carefully crafted and created to the best of the author's knowledge and personal experience. It comprises text templates and application guidelines for professional hypnosis sessions. The author is a licensed psychotherapist with extensive experience in psychotherapy, coaching, and personal training using hypnotic techniques and methods. Nevertheless, the author and the publisher assume no liability for the accuracy of information, instructions, and advice, nor for any typographical errors. The author and publisher accept no responsibility or liability for the application of these texts and recommendations with clients or patients, nor for any potential consequences or unexpected reactions. It is expressly noted that the application of therapeutic and advisory techniques and formulations lies solely and entirely within the responsibility of the practitioner. This also applies to adherence to the boundaries of legally regulated medical and therapeutic practices. The fact that a book containing action proposals is freely available for sale does not imply that its application with clients or patients is permitted for everyone.

Hypnosis 1

... ... You can open yourself up to meeting other people again ... ... because you know it's time to make new connections and overcome loneliness ... ... You can open yourself up to meeting other people again ... ... because you're truly ready now to take new paths ... ... You can open yourself up to meeting other people again ... ... because today you're engaging in self-reflection during this trance, and this trance will clear the way ... ... You can open yourself up to meeting other people again ... ... because in trance, you can change your inner perspective most easily to find new connections ... ... New encounters and new connections await you ... ...

... ... What you can imagine in your thoughts can become the next truth of your life ... ... and that's why you imagine yourself meeting friendly people ... ... What you can imagine in your thoughts can become the next truth of your life ... ... and that's why you imagine yourself finding new acquaintances and friends ... ... What you can imagine in your thoughts can become the next truth of your life ... ...

and that's why you now imagine how it will feel when you feel better ... ... What you can imagine in your thoughts can become the next truth of your life ... ... and that's why you imagine there are people waiting for you ... ... New encounters and new connections await you ... ...

... ... The relaxation of your body helps you to be and stay relaxed internally ... ... and that's why it's easy for you to let go of heavy thoughts ... ... The relaxation of your body helps you to be and stay relaxed internally ... ... and that's why you can feel comfortable in this calmness ... ... The relaxation of your body helps you to be and stay relaxed internally ... ... and that's why you can feel good even when you're alone ... ... The relaxation of your body helps you to be and stay relaxed internally ... ... and that's why you can approach everyday life with ease to discover new things ... ... New encounters and new connections await you ... ...

... ... You are always a friend to yourself, and you can meet yourself ... ... and with that, you create a strong connection ... ... You are always a friend to yourself, and you can meet yourself ... ... and with that, you overcome loneliness, even within yourself ... ... You are always a friend to yourself, and you can meet yourself ... ... and with that, there is always a way to be in contact ... ... You are always a friend to yourself, and you can meet yourself ... ... and in this self-encounter lies the opportunity for encounters with other people ... ... New encounters and new connections await you ... ...

... ... You open yourself up to your fellow human beings again and approach them ... ... You can do this because you've done it before ... ... You open yourself up to your fellow human beings again and approach them ... ... because this is the fastest way to overcome loneliness ... ... You open yourself up to your fellow human beings again and approach them ... ... because this is how you use your own strength and potential ... ... You open yourself up to your fellow human beings again and approach them ... ... because this is how you best realize that there are people waiting for new encounters, just like you ... ... New encounters and new connections await you ... ...

... ... You feel connected to yourself and the calm you feel now ... ... and this self-connection helps you to connect with others ... ... You feel connected to yourself and the calm you feel now ... ... and this self-connection dissolves loneliness ... ... You feel connected to yourself and the calm you feel now ... ... and this self-connection leads you out of loneliness and into new connections ... ... Loneliness fades away ... ... You feel connected ... ... You truly feel connected ... ...

Hypnosis 2

... ... You have a deep desire to overcome loneliness and feel good again ... ... Perhaps you can't easily change being alone ... ... But being alone doesn't have to mean being lonely ... ... Loneliness fades with activity, and if you could stand beside yourself and observe, you might say ... ... You accept the challenge ... ... You tackle it actively and overcome the feeling of loneliness with hypnosis ... ... because you could affirm it to yourself ... ... because you could say to yourself ... ... It's good that you're here, using this hypnosis ... ... Right now, in this trance, you can experience something special ... ... Now you're close to your feelings and not lonely at all ... ... so you can feel much more clearly what you really feel ... ... There are so many feelings behind loneliness ... ... Right now, you feel no loneliness ... ... so you can now find other feelings ... ... Imagine you could take this feeling and inner experience into your everyday life, thinking this way all the time; it would prove ... ... This hypnosis ends loneliness ... ... The suggestions help you develop inner freedom, openness, and contentment ... ...

... ... If you could freely choose what this hypnosis should accomplish, you might say ... ... Loneliness should end now ... ... because you want this difficult time to truly end, and you want to feel joy in life again ... ... You might also feel uncertain and think that it can't be that easy to be connected with others again ... ... Maybe you miss companionship or friendship, and you wonder how you can change it ... ... If the oppressive feeling of loneliness were to end, then you could feel ... ... Freedom and openness to new things arising deep within you ... ... Freedom and openness to new things lie in your thoughts and feelings ... ... Perhaps you have thought before ... ... Loneliness fades as soon as you open yourself to new things ... ... but then found that it wasn't so easy ... ... But it can succeed ... ... And when you succeed in overcoming loneliness, even if just once, you'll likely wish ... ... This is good, and this is how it should be ... ... Building the New ... ... Surely you've often heard it said ... ... Deep inside, you always find a friend ... ... or ... ... Deep within, you always find an ally ... ... But it's not always so easy to feel this in everyday life ...

… … … There were also times in your life when you were certain … … You truly feel trust and friendship … … because you had friends and trusted ones … … … … Maybe you were so well connected in acquaintanceships, friendships, and relationships before that you would have told a lonely person … … Reach out to others and trust in new and interesting encounters … … because it was easy for you at that time … … … … In this moment, you're accepting suggestions without thinking about them … … You're in a trance, so it's easy for you to say … … You are confident, and you confidently reach out to others … … and with that, loneliness passes … … … … And when you find it easier to connect with others in your waking life because the suggestions work and make it easy for you, then you experience success and suddenly see … … Friendships and relationships are always possible … … Maybe you'll experience this realization as soon as tomorrow or very soon; who knows … …

… … Suggestions work now and will continue to work later … … As soon as you feel the effects of the suggestions in your everyday life, you'll know for sure … … Loneliness is truly over … … and … … Your feeling toward yourself and others has changed ... ... And when you experience this and meet someone who feels lonely and seeks help, you might say to them ... ... Trust yourself ... ... because ... ... Inside, you'll always find a friend ... ... You might then say to this lonely person ... ... You'll see, when you're a friend to yourself, you'll find other friends too ... ... But you yourself will experience and assess what effects have occurred and what this hypnosis has changed and accomplished in you ... ... You'll come to your own decision ... ... You'll experience the effects of this hypnosis ... ... and then you can feel what has changed ... ... And after you've experienced that loneliness has passed, you might then repeatedly say with confidence to another ... ... The hypnosis has driven away the loneliness ... ... The suggestions help you discover connections and friendships ... ... Connection to yourself and friendship with others ... ... And anyone who follows this path can convince themselves of it ... ...

Hypnosis 3

... ... You want to finally overcome loneliness today ... ... You have this desire, this goal ... ... You want to connect with yourself and with others, and be in connection with yourself and others ... ... You want to reach out to others again and feel good ... ... You want to feel good even when you're alone because being alone does not mean being lonely ... ... So, accept the following suggestions and choose the ones you resonate with the most ... ... The suggestions you agree with will have the strongest effect ... [hidden memory of the previous session with hidden instructions] ... These are the best suggestions ... ...

... You accept ... the challenge ... [5-10 second pause] ... ... You approach this ... actively ... [5-10 second pause] ... ... You overcome ... the feeling of loneliness ... with hypnosis ... [5-10 second pause] ... ... Now you are ... close to your feelings ... and not lonely at all ... [5-10 second pause] ... ... Now ... you feel ... no loneliness ... [5-10 second pause] ... ... This ... hypnosis ... ends loneliness ... [5-10 second pause] ... ... The ... suggestions ... help you develop inner freedom ... [Now please pause for about 30 seconds] ...

... You accept ... the challenge ... [5-10 second pause] ... ... You approach this ... actively ... [5-10 second pause] ... ... You overcome ... the feeling of loneliness ... with hypnosis ... [5-10 second pause] ... ... Now you are ... close to your feelings ... and not lonely at all ... [5-10 second pause] ... ... Now ... you feel ... no loneliness ... [5-10 second pause] ... ... This ... hypnosis ... ends loneliness ... [5-10 second pause] ... ... The ... suggestions ... help you develop inner freedom ... [Now please pause for about 30 seconds] ...

... Loneliness ... should end now ... [5-10 second pause] ... ... Freedom and openness to new things arise ... deep within you ... [5-10 second pause] ... ... Freedom ... and openness are in your thoughts and feelings ... [5-10 second pause] ... ... Loneliness fades away as soon as you open yourself ... to new things ... [5-10 second pause] ... ... This is ... good ... and this is how it should be ... [Now please pause for about 30 seconds] ...

... Loneliness ... should end now ... [5-10 second pause] ... ... Freedom and openness to new things arise ... deep within you ... [5-10 second pause] ... ... Freedom ... and openness are in your thoughts and feelings ... [5-10 second pause] ... ... Loneliness fades away as soon as you open yourself ... to new things ... [5-10 second pause] ... ... This is ... good ... and this is how it should be ... [Now please pause for about 30 seconds] ...

... Deep within ... you always find a friend ... [5-10 second pause] ... ... Deep inside you ... you always find ... an ally ... [5-10 second pause] ... ... You truly feel trust and ... friendship ... [5-10 second pause] ... ... Reach out to others ... and trust ... [5-10 second pause] ... ... Confidently ... you approach others ... [Now please pause for about 30 seconds] ...

... Deep within ... you always find a friend ... [5-10 second pause] ... ... Deep inside you ... you always find ... an ally ... [5-10 second pause] ... ... You truly feel trust and ... friendship ... [5-10 second pause] ... ... Reach out to others ... and trust ... [5-10 second pause] ... ... Confidently ... you approach others ... [Now please pause for about 30 seconds] ...

Distribution, publication, and copying in any form are prohibited and subject to damages.

... Your feeling ... towards yourself has changed ... [5-10 second pause] ... ... Trust yourself, because within you ... you always find a friend ... [5-10 second pause] ... ... You experience the effect of this ... hypnosis ... [5-10 second pause] ... ... The ... suggestions help you ... discover connections ... [5-10 second pause] ... ... Connection to yourself and ... friendship ... with others ... [Now please pause for about 30 seconds] ...

... Your feeling ... towards yourself has changed ... [5-10 second pause] ... ... Trust yourself, because within you ... you always find a friend ... [5-10 second pause] ... ... You experience the effect of this ... hypnosis ... [5-10 second pause] ... ... The ... suggestions help you ... discover connections ... [5-10 second pause] ... ... Connection to yourself and ... friendship ... with others ... [Now please pause for about 30 seconds] ...

Copying, publishing, and sharing with third parties are only permitted with the written consent of the author. Please observe the notes on copyright and usage.

Hypnosis 4

... ... You're going deep into trance now, allowing your subconscious to open up completely ... ... This is how you overcome your shyness today and become open to people again ... ... You're ready to truly accept all the suggestions and let them unfold ... ... This is how you overcome your shyness today and become open to people again ... ... You mentally prepare yourself for openness and communication with the following suggestions ... ... This is how you overcome your shyness today and become open to people again ... ... You develop joy in meeting others with this hypnosis ... ... This is how you overcome your shyness today and become open to people again ... ...

... ... First, you mentally align yourself with openness and a desire for connection ... ... and that's why you're strong and brave enough to approach other people ... ... Thoughts can guide our feelings ... ... and that's why you're strong and brave enough to approach other people ... ... Thoughts can guide our behaviors ... ... and that's why you're strong and brave enough to approach other people ...

... ... Thoughts help us believe in ourselves ... ... and that's why you're strong and brave enough to approach other people ... ... You believe in yourself and are confident in your positive energy ... ...

... ... Your body can take on an upright and stable posture ... ... and that's why you also come across as likable and interesting to others ... ... Your body is already adopting this posture, even now in this trance ... ... and that's why you also come across as likable and interesting to others ... ... Your face is relaxed and ready to smile warmly ... ... and that's why you also come across as likable and interesting to others ... ... Your face is already relaxing and smiling now, in this trance ... ... and that's why you also come across as likable and interesting to others ... ... You believe in yourself and are confident in your positive energy ... ...

... ... You feel the desire to have more connections and relationships again ... ... and that's why you look forward to actively reaching out to others ... ... You remember the good times when you had plenty of social contacts and friendships ... ... and that's why you look forward to actively reaching out to others ... ... You know how good it feels to be connected ... ... and that's why you look forward to actively reaching out to others ... ... You feel connected to yourself now and want to be connected with others too ... ... and that's why you look forward to actively reaching out to others ... ... You believe in yourself and are confident in your positive energy ... ...

... ... You overcome your shyness and all inhibitions ... ... because you actively engage with others and find contact and communication with them ... ... With every contact you make with others, you become more open and confident ... ... because you actively engage with others and find contact and communication with them ... ... With every step you take toward others, you become more proud ... ... because you actively engage with others and find contact and communication with them ... ... With every step you take toward others, you believe in yourself more and more ... ... because you actively engage with others and find contact and communication with them ... ... You believe in yourself and are confident in your positive energy ... ...

... ... You have truly embraced the suggestions you've heard ... ... and that's why you're now open and brave and looking forward to meeting others ... ... All suggestions are now working deeper and becoming anchored in your subconscious ... ... and that's why you're now open and brave and looking forward to meeting others ... ... Even after this hypnosis, all the suggestions you've heard will continue to work ... ... and that's why you're now open and brave and looking forward to meeting others ... ... You believe in yourself and are confident in your positive energy ... ... You firmly believe in yourself, and you are truly confident in your positive energy ... ...

Hypnosis 5

You want to overcome your loneliness today ... ... You want to feel good in your life again ... ... Contact with others is helpful, but only if you are connected with yourself ... ... because loneliness only arises from a lack of connection to ourselves ... ... Today you will find a helpful thought ... ... Today you will find within yourself a thought that helps you feel connected ... ... If you live alone, you will still be alone after this hypnosis ... ... alone but no longer lonely ... ... alone, but connected with yourself ... ... You will achieve this today ... ... You will achieve it because you accept a special thought ... ...

Imagine you are lying on a very comfortable lounge chair, somewhere outside in nature ... ... It's a beautiful, sunny day, and you've gently fallen asleep in the warm sun, dreaming beautiful dreams ... ... maybe you're dreaming of a happy past ... ... or you're dreaming of a beautiful future, a wonderful vision of what could soon be ... ... and with the images of this beautiful dream, pleasant and beautiful feelings arise within you ... ... Perhaps you know that we only dream feelings ... ... and the images and scenes we see in dreams are thoughts and imaginations that match these feelings ... ... You are now dreaming a beautiful dream because you have beautiful feelings deep inside you ... ... Deep within, there are always beautiful feelings ... ... because these feelings were stored during beautiful times ... ... Let yourself drift in these beautiful dream images ... ... change them if you want ... ... Let them be beautiful and remain beautiful, because now you should relax like in your most beautiful dreams ... ...

Then you wake up and look directly into the bright blue sky ... ... You still feel the beautiful and pleasant feelings of the dream because shortly after waking up, we always feel the feelings we dreamed of ... ... You dreamed so beautifully that you wake up with a very pleasant feeling ... ... still feeling so wonderfully good and realizing that it is still broad daylight ... ... And you look directly into the bright blue summer sky ... ... A few small white clouds pass by, and you see writing in the sky ... ... In bold letters, something is written there ... ... The clouds move on so you can clearly see and read the words ... ... You can clearly see it, you can read it because it is your own thought that is written there

… … Up there in the bright blue sky, it says what you know deep within … … what you truly believe deep within … … Up there it says … …

I am deeply connected with myself and enjoy feeling myself. I am one with myself and enjoy this.

… [Read the affirmation slowly and a little louder than the previous text to emphasize it. Then pause for about 30 seconds before continuing to read.] …

Then you think about how often you have felt lonely and disconnected because you were alone … … You tried to find joy … … perhaps also to connect with others … … But often it was the case that you were still alone … … Being alone does not have to mean being lonely … … but over time, it has felt that way … … Even though it is nice to be in contact with others and to have loving people around us, there is also a deep connection to ourselves … … We can often be alone, but we are never lonely if we feel connected to ourselves … … Your thought connects you with yourself … … The thought that is written in the sky and is your own reminds you of this connection … … Your own thought reminds you that you are deeply connected with yourself …

... an unbreakable and strong connection to yourself ... ... a loyal and ever-present connection to yourself ... ... This is the most important connection ... ... because only self-connection can overcome loneliness ... ... only in self-connection can loneliness fade away ... ... Deep inside you, these words echo like a sound ... ... They catch you, because deep inside you, you are never alone and never lonely ... ... Once again, the words you hear resonate ... ...

I am deeply connected with myself and enjoy feeling myself. I am one with myself and enjoy this.

... [Read the affirmation slowly and a little louder than the previous text to emphasize it. Then pause for about 30 seconds before continuing to read.] ...

... ... These special words resonate deep within you and help you feel connected even without other people ... ... because you are always connected with yourself ... ... They help you be alone and still feel connected ... ... and to stay in this connection ... ...

Your affirmation helps you live in harmony with yourself again ... ... in connection with yourself ... ... in a connection that supports you, especially when you are alone ... ... And with each repetition of your affirmation, you can feel the connection to yourself more clearly ... ... You are never lonely within yourself ... ... You are never truly lonely because you are connected with yourself ... ...

Hypnosis 6

You've been feeling lonely for some time now ... ... You're alone, but being alone isn't the biggest problem ... ... What's difficult is that someone you loved deeply is no longer with you ... ... You've experienced a separation, and your heart is still attached to this connection ... ... You know you need to let go of this connection because it's over ... ... Perhaps not for you, as you haven't fully detached yet ... ... Letting go doesn't mean forgetting ... ... What the relationship once meant to you, and what it still means, can remain as a memory, an experience, and a feeling within you forever ... ... as a feeling that finds its place deep within you ... ... and you'll become open to the life you must now create without this person ... ... Today, in this trance, you can speak with an entity that can help you take this step ... ... Maybe you're religious and can pray ... ... to God or Jesus or an angel ... ... or you speak to yourself, believing that there is a deep inner strength that can and will help you ... ... your subconscious or your reflection ... ... You might say ... ...

Dear Self in the Mirror / Dear God / Dear Guardian Angel / Dear Subconscious ... ... I want to overcome loneliness ... ... I know I must continue living alone after this separation ... ... I must walk my path alone ... ... So, I want to try to let go and keep a good memory ... ... At the same time, I want to open myself up to life and allow new experiences ... ... I want to let go of holding on and clinging, and I ask you ... ... dear Self in the Mirror / dear God / dear Guardian Angel / dear Subconscious ... ... support me and show me the way to my inner center, where I will find the strength to overcome and let go ... ...

Dear Self in the Mirror / Dear God / Dear Guardian Angel / Dear Subconscious ... ... I know I must actively turn to life ... ... I know I can keep memories, but I mustn't stay stuck in them ... ... I want to open myself up to the beauty and risks of life again ... ... because the unpredictable makes life worth living ... ... I trust that you can help me with your guidance ... ... I trust that I can truly open myself up to new things again and recognize every day that I am worthy of leading a liberated life ... ... because with each step forward, I move out of loneliness ... ... I know I only feel lonely when I stand still and think about the past, holding onto memories

... ... With your help, I repeatedly realize that memories remain within me while I continue forward ... ... Dear Self in the Mirror / Dear God / Dear Guardian Angel / Dear Subconscious ... ... please support me in enjoying the time I spend with myself and spending it with a good feeling ... ... because only in this way can I find my inner center and begin my journey from there ... ...Dear Self in the Mirror / Dear God / Dear Guardian Angel / Dear Subconscious ... ... I'm fully aware that I need to take care of my feelings ... ... I want to allow all my feelings, especially the feeling of loneliness if it's truly there ... ... Often, I've felt lonely because I wished that he/she ... [Best to mention the name of the person the client had to part with] ... was still there ... ... I know that I may feel alone once I accept that this relationship is over, but not lonely ... ... With your help ... ... dear Self in the Mirror / dear God / dear Guardian Angel / dear Subconscious ... ... I understand well when I am lonely and when I am just alone and can look forward ... ...

Dear Self in the Mirror / Dear God / Dear Guardian Angel / Dear Subconscious ... ... Please help me quickly leave lonely moments behind if they do reoccur ... ... I know I need some time to fully let go and accept that this relationship is over and that I now live without him/her ... [Best to mention the name of the person the client had to part with] ... but I can do it ... ... I trust that you will also help me be patient with myself if this isn't as easy as I'd like it to be ... ... I thank you now for your support ... ... dear Self in the Mirror / dear God / dear Guardian Angel / dear Subconscious ... ...

Now, immerse yourself fully in your feelings and feel your inner center ... ... Trust entirely in your body's sensation that shows you the way to your inner center ... ... Breathe calmly and deeply in and out, and feel your center ... ... There lies your strength ... ... There, you will find help ... ... Every helping entity guides you there ... ... The support of your helper becomes self-help deep within you ... ... because deep inside you, there is always a helper ... [Please adjust the gender to match the client's] ... who has also been addressed by these words ... ... So, your inner self is ready to do everything it can to help you overcome loneliness and open up to new things ... ... There is always and everywhere your Self in the Mirror ... ...

Hypnosis 7

You want to end the time of loneliness ... ... You want to experience closeness and community again ... ... Belonging and love ... ... The starting point for any positive change is yourself ... ... Your closeness and love for yourself are the starting point for fulfilling contact and constructive relationships with others ... ...

... ... Today, you will find the greatest help for this ... ... In the state of trance, as comfortable and calm as you are right now, it is easy to find help within yourself ... ... in your subconscious ... ... much more help than in the waking state ... ...

Now you can talk to your subconscious and experience a truly positive change ... ... Your subconscious helps you because it hears and understands my words, which become your own ... ... You speak them internally with me ... ... So you yourself are the one who says ... ...

... ... I turn my gaze inward to perceive and accept my deepest feelings ... ... and my own deep feelings come to me openly and reveal themselves clearly and genuinely ... ... I dive deeper and deeper into my innermost self and let myself fall into the depths of my inner center ... ... and in my inner center, my thoughts and feelings catch me softly and safely ... ... I am happy that in this pleasant trance and silence, I can truly meet myself and learn new things about myself ... ... and my innermost self, the part of me that I cannot easily reach in the waking state, rejoices with me in this deep encounter ... ...

... ... I am now ready for a deep and honest encounter with myself, especially with the feeling of loneliness within me ... ... and I meet other people who are also ready to enter into honest and genuine relationships ... ... I accept myself and meet myself with interest and curiosity ... ... and I recognize more and more that others also meet me with honest interest and curiosity and are waiting for me ... ... I trust that I will become better and better at being a good friend to myself and feeling this self-connection ... ... and I experience friendship and connection in my encounters with other people ... ...

… … What I give to myself returns positively to my life … … What I give to myself and to others, my fellow human beings give to themselves and also to me … …

… … I look forward to meeting other people, and I go through my daily life with open eyes and a smile … … and just as openly and friendly, many people who are smiling also meet me every day … … … … I approach my fellow human beings with an open heart and sincere interest … … and everywhere, I meet open people who are interested in sincere interaction and open their hearts … …

… … I trust my fellow human beings because I feel who is genuine, and because I know there are no guarantees … … and with trust and honesty, my fellow human beings approach me and are happy about spending time together … …

… … I feel very clearly that I am a true friend to myself with my positive thoughts and my attention to myself … … and I experience friendship in my encounters with others every day … … … … I accept myself every day and meet myself with interest and curiosity … … and every day, interesting people approach me and meet me with interest and curiosity ... ...

... ... I am an enrichment for my fellow human beings, and with joy, I bring meaning to their lives ... ... and my fellow human beings are an enrichment for me, and with joy, they bring meaning to my life ... ...

Hypnosis 8

You're fighting against loneliness ... ... But it's time to end this fight ... ... Loneliness is not an enemy; it's a feeling ... ... All feelings have a reason and make sense ... ... Feelings show us what is happening inside us ... ... Farewells or times when we are often and long alone show up as a feeling of inner emptiness ... ... in a longing that we cannot easily fulfill ... ... This then leads to loneliness, which fades away when we accept and appreciate it as our feeling ... ... When we accept this feeling and understand that it belongs to us and shows us that something is missing, it can already pass because we can set out to discover new things and find what we're missing ... ... It's never an object or a person that we absolutely need ... ... We can miss people deeply and suffer from separations, but what we miss is closeness ... ... or togetherness ... ... Familiarity or security ... ... Understanding and closeness ... ... Perhaps you miss a completely different feeling, but it's always feelings that we're missing, which then manifest as loneliness ... ... As soon as you accept loneliness, it fades away, and your true needs reveal themselves behind it ... ... Sometimes we get stuck and only feel loneliness ... ... That's how it happened ... ... But behind loneliness, your deep needs are waiting for you ... ... As soon as you accept loneliness, your needs reveal themselves, and you can look forward again and find ways to fulfill them ... ... Feelings also show up in our bodies ... ... So today, you can use your body's perception and your body's feelings to accept loneliness and thus end it ... ... You can do it ... ... It's truly possible, and you'll succeed today ... ... It succeeds today ... ... It succeeds today ... ...

Now feel your body ... ... become consciously and clearly aware of it ... ... Feel what your body feels ... ... Feel the calm and relaxation ... ... Let your body become even calmer, so you can feel the feelings it shows you even better ... ... Somewhere in your body, there is also the feeling of loneliness now ... ... perhaps it's very faint now ... ... almost like a memory because you feel good now ... ... But loneliness has its place and is there ... ... maybe as a gut feeling in the middle of your body ... ... or as a feeling in your heart ... ... possibly also in a completely different place, because every single cell in your body knows your feelings ... ... the loneliness, but also all the feelings behind it ... ...

all the needs that are important now and want to be seen by you ... ... needs that can be fulfilled ... ... maybe for contact or for trust ... ... who knows ... ... maybe for self-connection and self-care ... ... Now find the spot on your body where you can feel the loneliness best ... ... or, if you can't really grasp it now, the spot where you most expect loneliness to be ... ... and focus on this spot ... ... Imagine that loneliness is sitting there ... ... or that it was sitting there when it was particularly strong ... ... If you want and if it's possible, you can now place your hand there ... ... place a hand on your body ... ... on your stomach or on your heart or wherever the loneliness might be ... ... Feel this spot and accept the loneliness ... ... Accept it as a signal for something more important ... ... Accept it as a signal for your needs ... ... for needs that you can recognize even better the more you focus on this spot ... ... You accept loneliness, and it fades away ... ... and behind the loneliness, your true needs reveal themselves, which you can feel now ... ... You feel your true needs now ... ... Also accept these needs, because with them comes a new feeling that you can feel in a few moments ... ... in the same spot ... ... Loneliness fades away, and a new feeling emerges there ... ... More and more, the feeling of the new emerges ... ... the desire for a fresh start ... ... the impulse of a new beginning ... ... By accepting loneliness, your true needs, which are very different ... ... different from loneliness ... ... By accepting loneliness, the feeling of the new also reveals itself ... ... the impulse to start anew ... ... These are the feelings that are truly within you, and your body shows them to you ... ... The more you succeed in concentrating on the spot you found on your body and feeling your body there ... ... the more you succeed in feeling your true needs ... ... or just letting them quietly work for you ... ... You don't have to be able to name them ... ... Just allow them, as you allowed loneliness ... ... Then, more and more, you can feel the inner breakthrough ... ... Imagine that where all this is happening in your body, where you feel it, there is a small sun shining inside your body ... ... a small sun that gives you warmth, strength, and confidence for this breakthrough ... ... Let this warming sun grow larger with each breath ... ... This way, your entire body is informed ... ... Your whole body is informed about the inner breakthrough ... ... The time of loneliness is over ... ... You feel good and look forward to your breakthrough ... ... You look forward to the new ... ... Your whole body is informed that loneliness fades away and is replaced by the impulses of inner breakthrough ... ... Every cell in your body knows that now is the time for inner breakthrough ... ... Time for new paths ... ... Time for new encounters ... ... time for you ... ...

Keep breathing calmly and evenly and trust that your body feels more inner warmth with each further breath ... ... Trust that with each further breath, loneliness fades away, if it's still there at all ... ... Loneliness ends ... ... over and over again because now is the time for your true needs ... ... Now is the time for inner warmth ... ... Now is the time for inner breakthrough ... ... Now is the time for new beginnings ... ... Now your time begins ... ... Now your time begins ... ...

Hypnosis 9

Instructions for Implementation

In this hypnosis, a self-hypnosis trigger will be established. A self-hypnosis trigger is a signal that initiates the state of trance. With its help, even an inexperienced client can continue to practice self-hypnosis at home. They can work with simple suggestions that they can easily remember and that we should prepare, or even with simple visualizations. Triggered self-hypnosis is a very good tool to give the client a task and to support the therapy. This way, the time between appointments in the practice is not without therapy but is continued at home. A completely self-controlled self-hypnosis without a trigger is also learnable but requires a lot of time and practice. Establishing the trigger is a fairly simple task and naturally relieves the client, as I do not want to burden them with training self-controlled self-hypnosis. Despite all the naysayers, I also claim here that there is really no problem in teaching a client a simple trigger self-hypnosis. It is no more dangerous than meditation, autogenic training, or yoga. You survive those at home unscathed too. I have experienced numerous patients in my practice who not only managed well with self-hypnosis but also enjoyed it. And if a patient likes to do self-hypnosis, no matter how simple the suggestion may look, then that is a very good support for compliance. Discuss the procedure once before hypnosis and give the client a short, keyword-based list of the steps of self-hypnosis so that they have a small guide.

+++ End of Instructions +++

Sometimes you feel lonely when you're alone ... ... Then it's not always easy to get out of that feeling ... ... Self-hypnosis can help you overcome the most difficult moments and quickly achieve a feeling of connection ... ... Because with self-hypnosis, you can feel much better than in the waking state that you are so deeply connected with yourself deep inside that you cannot feel any loneliness deep within your feeling ... ... So you can let go of the feeling of loneliness even when there's no one who can be with you ... ... It's actually quite simple, and I'll show you how to do it ...

... You'll learn how to do it now ... ... now you're in trance, so you can now also easily learn to do self-hypnosis ... ...

I'll show you how to initiate trance ... ... There's a trigger, a code word that brings you into trance ... ... It is ... ... Ridola ... [Please emphasize the made-up word on the "Ri" ... Ri-dola.] ... ... Make yourself comfortable at home and close your eyes, just like here ... ... and then whisper this trigger over and over again until you become tired, and that happens quickly ... ... You'll become very tired very quickly when you whisper ... ... Ridola – Ridola –Ridola - Ridola – Ridola –Ridola ... ... and in doing so, you'll already achieve a pleasant trance, just like here ... ... Your trigger ... ... Ridola ... ... is now deeply imprinted in your subconscious ... ... So you can simply use it whenever you want to enter trance ... ...

Then you go deeper into trance because in a deeper trance, there is no feeling of loneliness ... ... In a deep trance, you are very close to yourself, and this closeness leaves no room for loneliness ... ... You enter this deeper trance by whispering ten times ... ... I go deeper and deeper, towards calm ... ... You simply whisper ... ... I go deeper and deeper, towards calm ... ... I go once deeper and deeper, towards calm ... ... I go twice deeper and deeper, towards calm ... ... I go three times deeper and deeper, towards calm, and so on ... ... until you finally reach ten and whisper ... ... I go ten times deeper and deeper, towards calm ... ... and in doing so, you enter this deeper trance, where you never feel lonely but always connected ... ... connected with yourself ... ... The trance you reach is deep and pleasant, just like here ... ... You are in complete safety ... ...

Then comes the main part of your self-hypnosis ... ... The main part helps you especially to turn the feeling of loneliness, when it's particularly strong, into a feeling of connection ... ... Connection with yourself, because you are always there ... ... You work in this part with a suggestion that frees you ... ... You simply whisper it ten times in a row ... ... Ten times, you whisper ... ... I find security and peace deep within me ... ... You count again ... ... You say ... ... I find security and peace deep within me once ... ... I find security and peace deep within me twice ... ... I find security and peace deep within me three times ... ... I find security and peace deep within me ten times ... ... and then you feel that you are never lonely inside ... ... You feel connected to yourself and to your memories ... ...To wake yourself up again, imagine a cold wind blowing ... ... Then you say ... ... I will wake up now and feel good ... ... and then you count out loud and clearly to three and open your eyes ... ... It's very easy ... ... So, once again ... ... To wake up again, imagine a cold wind blowing and say ... ... I will wake up now and feel good – One – Two – Three ... ... and then open your eyes because you're awake ... ... It's very easy, and you can try it later ... ...

You now know how self-hypnosis works ... ... You can use it from now on when you feel particularly lonely, to quickly feel a sense of connection again, where loneliness fades away because it's no longer possible ... ... You've learned how to quickly enter trance with your trigger and you know how to proceed ... ... Your trigger, Ridola, brings you into trance, which you deepen with the words ... ... I go deeper and deeper, towards calm ... ... Then follows your suggestion ... ... I find security and peace deep within me ... This suggestion dispels loneliness ... ... At the end of self-hypnosis, you then imagine a cold wind and say ... I will wake up now and feel good – One – Two – Three ... ...

Hypnosis 10

There's a place deep inside you where you can never be alone ... ... It's a place where you are always connected with yourself and always find yourself ... ... At this place, you can change everything ... ... Your breathing leads you there ... ... Imagine you could leave your body with your breath, like a spirit for whom there are no boundaries ... ... In your imagination, it's possible, it's even easy ... ... So, with the wind of your breath, you leave your body and move freely and lightly ... ... letting yourself drift through space and time ... ... letting yourself fall deeper and deeper into your own creativity and imagination, which both lie deep in your feeling ... ... There you reach this special place that awaits you ... ... the land of your dreams ... ... And with the next breath, you arrive in the land of dreams ... ...

You're standing in a beautiful landscape, probably the most beautiful you've ever seen ... ... and you take a deep breath in and out and take in the scent of fresh flowers ... ... You're standing in a meadow, and everywhere, radiant flowers are blooming, smelling wonderful ... ... a landscape to dream in ... ... So, you start walking, step by step, calmly across this flower meadow, and you think about the feeling of loneliness ... ... Often, you've felt it, felt so alone and also lonely ... ... Being alone doesn't automatically mean being lonely ... ... In such a quiet and beautiful landscape, you can be alone and feel good, maybe even enjoy being alone ... ... That has certainly often been the case in your everyday life ... ... Conversely, it can happen that we are not alone at all, maybe even surrounded by people most of the time, and still feel lonely ... ... or perhaps precisely because of that ... ... because despite this apparent closeness to other people or to a specific person, there is no real sense of togetherness or belonging ... ... We can be lonely ... ... even in contact with others ... ... But the worst loneliness we feel is when we lose ourselves ... ... when we are no longer connected to ourselves ... ... This too is possible in waking life ... ... We can lose ourselves, at least in our perception, in our thinking and actions ... ... In the land of dreams, we never lose ourselves ... ... Here we always find ourselves ... ... Here we always meet ourselves ... ... because everything here is you ... ... You yourself are the flower meadow ... ... You yourself are every blossom ... ... You yourself are the ground you walk on here ... ... You see in front of you a huge glass ball ... ... It lies in the middle of the flower meadow, and you go towards it ... ... It's the ball of the one moment ... ... It's called that because in this ball, in the land of dreams, you can change everything in a single moment ... ... because in a single moment, you can learn something about yourself that you didn't know before ... ... something that positively changes your life ... ... You approach the ball ... ... And because there are no boundaries for you in the land of dreams, you step inside the ball ... ... That's possible with a single step ... ... and you take that step now ... ... You stand in the ball and still think about the feeling of loneliness ... ... and while you're thinking, images form by themselves, showing themselves on the inner walls of the ball ... ... Images that appear like film clips on the wall of the ball ... ... You might first see images of situations where you felt particularly lonely or still feel lonely ... ... Maybe you see yourself alone ... ... You're thinking, brooding ... ... or you're doing something to distract yourself ... ... Maybe you're just waiting for time to pass ... ... Perhaps you also see images and scenes that show you together with other people ... ... But you still feel lonely or maybe even precisely because of that ... ... because no real connection is being made ... ... or because you're missing something that you can't get from these people ... ... It could also be that several images alternate and then a very special person appears ... ... on the glass wall of the ball of the one moment ... ... deep within you ... ... in your feelings ... ... in the land of dreams ... ... This one person might have the most to do with your loneliness ... ... Maybe you miss them ... ... because they're no longer with you ... ... because there was a separation ... ... or because this person no longer lives ... ... Then it might have been grief that you couldn't properly process and that you still feel as loneliness today ... ... Maybe an image of a still-living person comes to mind, someone who even lives with you ... ... and yet you sometimes feel lonely ... ... Let all the images that come to mind or simply appear before your inner eye be there, and accept them ... ... Let them be there because they belong to you ... ... They show you a part of your loneliness ... ... You don't have to do anything now; just look at the images, because in doing so, deep within you, you learn to accept loneliness as a feeling and to reconcile yourself with it ... ... It has tormented you, and you have suffered, but today, in the land of dreams, it is possible to recognize loneliness as a part of yourself and to let it be there because they are helping images that you are looking at ... ... because by allowing these images and memories, something special happens within you ... ... A connection arises, or more precisely, a connection renews itself, which is the most important ... ... the connection to yourself ... ... So often, you have taken care of others and the relationship with other people that you eventually thought you could only experience yourself by being with others ... ... But the land of dreams tells you that it's the other way around ... ... When you're connected with yourself, then you can also enter into a constructive contact with others ... ... Connected with yourself, you can experience and shape beautiful relationships ... ... This connection with yourself is now being created, is now being reactivated and renewed, because within it, you can never be lonely ... ... You look at the glass wall and see your reflection ... ... Let it be there ... ... Accept it because it's the most important image ... ...

Trusting that you are connecting more and more with yourself internally, accepting yourself more and more, you step out of the ball, taking a step outside ... ... You stand on the flower meadow, and your reflection unfolds more and more inside the ball ... ... You walk further, step by step ... ... You walk towards the horizon because that's where your future begins ... ... and the future begins with the next breath ... ... On your way, you remind yourself that the land of dreams lies deep within you ... ... It has always been there ... ... I'm just telling you about it ... ...

Distribution, publication, and copying in any form are prohibited and subject to damages.

All Titles in the Series

Volume 1: Smoking Cessation
Volume 2: Anxiety and Restlessness
Volume 3: Burnout
Volume 4: Reducing Overweight
Volume 5: Coping with the Past
Volume 6: Suicidal Thoughts and Attempts
Volume 7: Psycho-Oncology
Volume 8: Obsessions and Tics
Volume 9: Self-Confidence and Decision-Making
Volume 10: Grief Work
Volume 11: Psychosomatics
Volume 12: Chronic Pain
Volume 13: Depressive Thoughts
Volume 14: Panic Attacks
Volume 15: Domestic Violence, Victim Support
Volume 16: Post-Traumatic Stress
Volume 17: Exam Anxiety and Stage Fright
Volume 18: Anti-Violence Training, Offender Support
Volume 19: Addiction Tendencies
Volume 20: Social Phobia and Fear of Contact
Volume 21: Nail Biting
Volume 22: Self-Awareness and Self-Love
Volume 23: Teeth Grinding and Night Clenching
Volume 24: Feelings of Guilt
Volume 25: Fear in Crowds
Volume 26: Fear of Flying, Aviophobia
Volume 27: Fear in Enclosed Spaces, Claustrophobia
Volume 28: Tinnitus, Ear Noises
Volume 29: Fear of Heights
Volume 30: Neurodermatitis

Copying, publishing, and sharing with third parties are only permitted with the written consent of the author. Please observe the notes on copyright and usage.

Volume 31: Finding Inner Balance
Volume 32: Overcoming Loneliness
Volume 33: Fear of Illness, Hypochondria
Volume 34: Anticipatory Anxiety, Fear of Fear
Volume 35: Jealousy in Relationships
Volume 36: Driving Anxiety
Volume 37: New Start after Separation
Volume 38: Fear of Injections
Volume 39: Heart Anxiety Neurosis
Volume 40: Overcoming Resentment and Anger
Volume 41: Resolving Blockages and Positive Thinking
Volume 42: Stress Reduction, Stress Management
Volume 43: Body Relaxation
Volume 44: Deep Relaxation
Volume 45: Fear of the Dark
Volume 46: Falling Asleep and Staying Asleep
Volume 47: Compulsive Buying
Volume 48: Restless Legs Syndrome
Volume 49: Bulimia
Volume 50: Anorexia
Volume 51: Overcoming Nightmares
Volume 52: Imagined Deformity
Volume 53: Overcoming Distrust, Finding Trust
Volume 54: Processing Failures
Volume 55: Humiliation, Emotional Hurt
Volume 56: Distressing Compassion, Vicarious Suffering
Volume 57: Self-Forgiveness
Volume 58: Self-Awareness, Self-Confidence
Volume 59: Saying No
Volume 60: Assertiveness
Volume 61: Setting Boundaries and Self-Assertion
Volume 62: Decision-Making Ability

Volume 63: Success Orientation
Volume 64: Ruminating, Circular Thinking
Volume 65: Accepting Pregnancy
Volume 66: Birth Preparation
Volume 67: Spiritual Opening
Volume 68: Joy of Life and Inner Lightness
Volume 69: Patience and Inner Peace
Volume 70: Fibromyalgia and Rheumatism
Volume 71: Irritable Bowel Syndrome, Crohn's Disease
Volume 72: Fear of Nausea, Emetophobia
Volume 73: Stuttering and Cluttering, Speech Flow Disorders
Volume 74: Concentration and Knowledge Anchoring
Volume 75: Vitality and Spontaneity
Volume 76: Searching for Meaning and Finding Goals
Volume 77: Life Crises, Life Events
Volume 78: Workaholism, Goal Obsession
Volume 79: Helper Syndrome, Helpless Helpers
Volume 80: Medication Abuse
Volume 81: Gambling Addiction
Volume 82: Internet Addiction, Smartphone Addiction
Volume 83: Hoarding Disorder, Compulsive Collecting
Volume 84: Conspiracy Thoughts, Overvalued Ideas
Volume 85: Fear of Operations and Treatments
Volume 86: Fear of Aging
Volume 87: Travel Anxiety
Volume 88: Anxiety When Urinating, Paruresis
Volume 89: Fear of Intimacy and Togetherness
Volume 90: Fear of Blushing
Volume 91: Coming Out in Homosexuality
Volume 92: Charisma Training
Volume 93: Migraines and Chronic Headaches
Volume 94: Overcoming Allergies, Bronchial Asthma

Volume 95: Normalizing Blood Pressure
Volume 96: Compulsive Perfectionism
Volume 97: Sports Hypnosis, Motivation
Volume 98: Sports Hypnosis, Performance Enhancement
Volume 99: Determination and Focus
Volume 100: Encountering the Inner Child
Volume 101: Cravings, Binge Eating
Volume 102: Stimulating Metabolism
Volume 103: Bipolar Mood Swings
Volume 104: Borderline, Identity Crises
Volume 105: Hypomania, Euphoria, Mania
Volume 106: Restlessness, Agitation
Volume 107: Nervous Breakdown
Volume 108: Adjustment Disorders
Volume 109: Self-Alienation, Depersonalization
Volume 110: Ending Self-Pity
Volume 111: Primary Gain of Illness
Volume 112: Secondary Gain of Illness
Volume 113: Bullying, Victim Support
Volume 114: Letting Go of Envy and Jealousy
Volume 115: Fear of Spiders, Arachnophobia
Volume 116: Fear of Dogs or Cats
Volume 117: Fear of Strangers, Xenophobia
Volume 118: Excessive Worries, Generalized Anxiety
Volume 119: Strengthening Sense of Responsibility
Volume 120: Unrequited Love, Heartache
Volume 121: Work-Life Balance
Volume 122: Letting Go of Unattainable Goals
Volume 123: Allowing and Accepting Help
Volume 124: Letting Go of Adult Children
Volume 125: Tourette Syndrome
Volume 126: Life Changes and New Starts

Volume 127: Accepting Life in a Wheelchair
Volume 128: Understanding and Overcoming Homesickness
Volume 129: Understanding and Overcoming Wanderlust
Volume 130: Dizziness, Meniere's Disease
Volume 131: Overcoming Aggression
Volume 132: Cutting and Self-Harm
Volume 133: Hair Pulling, Trichotillomania
Volume 134: Postpartum Depression
Volume 135: For Relatives of Dementia Patients
Volume 136: Self-Harm, Artificial Disorders
Volume 137: Activating Self-Healing Powers
Volume 138: Preventing Depression Relapse
Volume 139: Reactive Psychoses, Follow-Up
Volume 140: Obsessive Thoughts and Impulses
Volume 141: Compulsive Checking
Volume 142: Compulsive Counting, Symmetry Obsession
Volume 143: Compulsive Washing, Cleanliness Obsession
Volume 144: Compulsive Questioning
Volume 145: Dissociative Paralysis
Volume 146: Phantom Pain
Volume 147: Overcoming Complaining
Volume 148: Hay Fever, Pollen Allergy
Volume 149: Sexual Abuse, Victim Support
Volume 150: Standing Strong Against Sexism, #metoo
Volume 151: Binge Eating
Volume 152: Overcoming Thoughts of Revenge
Volume 153: Detachment from the Aggressor, Stockholm Syndrome
Volume 154: Courage to Separate
Volume 155: Chronic Fatigue, Exhaustion
Volume 156: Fear of the Future, Existential Anxiety
Volume 157: Excessive Worry About Children
Volume 158: Fear of Failure

Volume 159: Ending Distrust and Control
Volume 160: Dejection, Dysphoria
Volume 161: Boreout, Chronic Boredom
Volume 162: Bipolar Disorders, Relapse Prevention
Volume 163: Mania, Relapse Prevention
Volume 164: Nihilism, Feelings of Worthlessness
Volume 165: Thumb Sucking
Volume 166: Being Brave
Volume 167: Being Proud
Volume 168: Overcoming Shyness
Volume 169: Being Able to Delegate Responsibility
Volume 170: Being Able to Show Emotions
Volume 171: Letting Go of Guilt, Victim Support
Volume 172: Processing Guilt, Offender Support
Volume 173: Mood Swings, Cyclothymia
Volume 174: Lack of Drive, Vital Sadness
Volume 175: Hearing Voices with Reality Reference
Volume 176: Confident Communication
Volume 177: Standing Up for Oneself
Volume 178: Taking New Paths
Volume 179: Confident Job Application
Volume 180: No Longer Being Taken Advantage Of
Volume 181: End of Submissiveness
Volume 182: Depressive Numbness
Volume 183: Mood Drops, Affective Incontinence
Volume 184: Mood Instability
Volume 185: Somatoform Disorders
Volume 186: Stomach Ulcer, Psychosomatic
Volume 187: Accepting Amputation
Volume 188: Overcoming and Letting Go of Hatred
Volume 189: Ending Accusations
Volume 190: Allowing Tears, Being Able to Cry

Volume 191: Finding and Sorting Repressed Feelings
Volume 192: Somatoform Pain
Volume 193: Living Autonomously
Volume 194: Anhedonia, Joylessness
Volume 195: Persistent Sadness
Volume 196: Obesity, Food Addiction
Volume 197: Parents of Abused Children
Volume 198: Letting Go and Letting Be
Volume 199: Childhood Sexual Abuse
Volume 200: Fear of Loss

www.ingramcontent.com/pod-product-compliance
Lightning Source LLC
Chambersburg PA
CBHW030507220526
45464CB00006B/2694